Extreme Survival Medicine & First Aid

Mastering Vital Skills for Emergencies | Survival Medicine & First Aid

Lizzie Black

Survival Medicine & First Aid
© Copyright 2023 by Lizzie Black
All rights reserved

TABLE OF CONTENTS

Chapter 1: Assessing the Situation

Evaluating the Severity of an Emergency

Identifying Immediate Threats to Safety

Formulating a Quick Action Plan

Chapter 2: Building Your First Aid Kit

Essential Supplies for a Well-Equipped Kit

Tailoring Your Kit to Specific Needs

Maintaining and Updating Your Supplies

Chapter 3: Basic First Aid Skills

Handling Cuts, Burns, and Abrasions

Treating Fractures and Sprains

Managing Shock and Performing CPR:

Chapter 4: Wilderness First Aid

Navigating Medical Emergencies in the Great Outdoors

Dealing with Environmental Hazards

Utilizing Natural Resources for Survival

Chapter 5: Medical Emergencies

Identifying and Addressing Common Health Crises

Dealing with Allergies, Heart Attacks, and Strokes

Administering Medications When Necessary

Chapter 6: Injuries and Trauma

Techniques for Wound Care and Infection Prevention

Stopping Severe Bleeding

Handling Head Injuries and Spinal Trauma

Chapter 7: Survival Medicine for Specific Environments

Urban Survival Medicine

Rural Survival Medicine

Wilderness Survival Medicine

Travel Medicine

Chapter 8: Self-Care and Mental Resilience

Managing Stress and Anxiety in Survival Situations

Prioritizing Self-Care for Physical and Mental Well-Being

Fostering Resilience and Adaptability

Chapter 9: Communicating in Crisis

Effective Communication with Responders

Using Emergency Communication Devices

Conveying Medical Information Accurately

Chapter 10: Long-Term Survival Medicine

Sustaining Health and Hygiene over Extended Periods

Utilizing Natural Remedies and Herbal Medicine

Addressing Nutritional Needs during Survival Scenarios

Chapter 11: Community and Mutual Aid

The Power of Collaboration During Crises

Building a Support Network for Survival

Sharing Knowledge and Resources

Chapter 12: Preparing for the Unknown

Recognizing the Unpredictability of Emergencies

Constantly Updating Your Survival Skills

Encouraging Others to Prioritize Survival Education

CHAPTER 1: ASSESSING THE SITUATION

In the realm of survival medicine and first aid, the ability to assess a situation accurately and swiftly is akin to having a compass in the wilderness—it guides your actions and decisions, increasing your chances of success and survival. This chapter will serve as your compass, teaching you the critical skills needed to navigate the complex landscape of emergencies.

Evaluating the Severity of an Emergency

Imagine finding yourself in a scenario where someone is injured, or you are facing a challenging situation. The first step is to assess the severity of the emergency. But how do you do this?

Begin by observing the scene and gathering information. Look for clues like the number of people involved, the nature of injuries, and the presence of potential hazards. Is it a minor incident or a life-threatening crisis?

Learn how to categorize emergencies into different levels of severity. Is it a minor first aid situation, a moderate injury, or a critical emergency that requires immediate attention? This initial evaluation will dictate your next steps.

Identifying Immediate Threats to Safety

Safety is paramount during an emergency. To provide aid effectively, you must first ensure your own and others' safety. Here, we'll explore how to identify and mitigate immediate threats:

Understand the common dangers that can arise in various situations, such as fires, structural collapses, or environmental hazards.

Learn how to make quick decisions to remove yourself and others from harm's way. This may involve moving to a safer location, putting out a fire, or stabilizing a hazardous material.

Discover strategies for creating a safe zone around the emergency site. This ensures the safety of both victims and first responders.

Formulating a Quick Action Plan

Once you've assessed the situation's severity and secured the immediate safety of everyone involved, it's time to create a structured action plan:

Prioritize tasks based on the severity of injuries or needs. Learn the art of triage and how to allocate your resources efficiently.

Organize your response team, if available, and communicate the plan clearly. Effective teamwork is essential during emergencies.

Prepare for any necessary equipment, tools, or resources you might need. Having a well-equipped first aid kit and knowing how to use it can make a significant difference.

Chapter 2: Building Your First Aid Kit

In the realm of emergency preparedness, few tools are as vital as a well-organized and fully-stocked first aid kit. Whether you're at home, on the road, or venturing into the great outdoors, having the right supplies at your fingertips can be a lifesaver.

Essential Supplies for a Well-Equipped Kit

A properly equipped first aid kit should cover a range of common injuries and medical situations. Here's a breakdown of some essential supplies to consider:

- Bandages and Dressings: Assorted adhesive bandages, sterile gauze pads, and adhesive tape are fundamental for covering wounds and stopping bleeding.
- Antiseptics: Items like hydrogen peroxide, antiseptic wipes, and antibiotic ointment help prevent infection.
- Tools: Scissors, tweezers, and a thermometer are versatile tools for various medical tasks.
- Medications: Include over-the-counter pain relievers, antihistamines, and any prescription medications needed by family members.
- Personal Protective Equipment (PPE): Gloves, face masks, and eye protection are essential for infection control.
- Emergency Items: A digital thermometer, emergency blanket, and a CPR face shield should also be in your kit.

Tailoring Your Kit to Specific Needs

Consider the unique needs of your family, activities, and environment when customizing your first aid kit:

- Family-Specific Items: If you have children or elderly family members, include items like child-safe medications and supplies for managing age-related conditions.
- Activity-Based Supplies: Tailor your kit for specific activities such as hiking, camping, or boating. Insect repellent, snakebite kits, or motion sickness medication might be necessary.
- Allergies and Chronic Conditions: If anyone in your family has allergies, asthma, diabetes, or other chronic conditions, ensure you have the necessary supplies and medications.
- Location: The climate and environment where you live or travel can impact your kit. In cold regions, include items like hand warmers, while

in hot areas, sunblock and extra water may be critical.

Maintaining and Updating Your Supplies

A first aid kit is not a "set it and forget it" item. Regular maintenance is crucial:

- Check for Expiration Dates: Medications, ointments, and some supplies have expiration dates. Replace them as needed.

- Inspect for Damage: Make sure no items have leaked, deteriorated, or become damaged.

- Update for Changing Needs: As your family changes or your activities evolve, update your kit accordingly. This ensures you're always prepared for the specific situations you may encounter.

- Checklist and Inventory: Maintain a checklist of all items in your first aid kit. Periodically go through it to ensure everything is present and in good condition.

CHAPTER 3: BASIC FIRST AID SKILLS

Emergencies can happen suddenly and unexpectedly. Being equipped with basic first aid skills can make all the difference in providing immediate care and potentially saving a life. In this chapter, we'll explore fundamental first aid techniques for handling common injuries and medical emergencies.

Handling Cuts, Burns, and Abrasions

- Cuts and Lacerations: When faced with a cut, your immediate goal is to control bleeding.

Begin by cleaning the wound with soap and water. Apply gentle pressure with a sterile bandage or cloth. Elevate the injured area if possible. If bleeding persists, seek professional medical help.

- Burns: Burns are categorized into three levels: first-degree (superficial), second-degree (partial thickness), and third-degree (full thickness). First-degree burns typically involve redness and mild pain and can be treated with cold water and over-the-counter pain relievers. Second and third-degree burns require immediate medical attention.

- Abrasions (Scrapes): Clean the area with soap and water to prevent infection. Apply an over-the-counter antibiotic ointment and cover the abrasion with a sterile dressing. Keep the wound clean and monitor for signs of infection.

Treating Fractures and Sprains

- Fractures: If you suspect a fracture, immobilize the injured area to prevent further damage. Use splints, rolled-up newspapers, or available materials to support the injured limb. Do not attempt to realign the bones. Seek professional medical help promptly.

- Sprains: Rest, ice, compression, and elevation (RICE) are the key principles in treating sprains. Rest the injured area, apply ice to reduce swelling, use compression bandages to support the injury, and elevate the limb to minimize swelling.

Managing Shock and Performing CPR:

- Shock: Shock is a life-threatening condition that can result from various injuries or medical emergencies. Symptoms include rapid, shallow breathing, a weak pulse, and altered mental state. Lay the person down with their feet elevated if possible. Cover them with a blanket and reassure them until medical help arrives.

- Cardiopulmonary Resuscitation (CPR): CPR is a critical skill for reviving someone who has stopped breathing or whose heart has stopped. The American Heart Association recommends the hands-only CPR technique for untrained individuals. Call 911, then place your hands in the center of the chest and push hard and fast to the beat of the classic disco song "Stayin' Alive" (about 100-120 compressions per minute).

By mastering these basic first aid skills, you'll be better prepared to respond to common injuries and emergencies. However, it's important to remember that first aid is not a replacement for professional medical care. In severe cases or when in doubt, always seek immediate medical attention.

CHAPTER 4: WILDERNESS FIRST AID

When venturing into the wilderness, whether for a weekend camping trip or an extended backcountry excursion, being prepared for medical emergencies is paramount. In remote areas, access to immediate medical care is limited, and self-reliance becomes crucial. This chapter explores the unique challenges of wilderness first aid, including navigating medical emergencies in the great outdoors, dealing with environmental hazards, and utilizing natural resources for survival.

Navigating Medical Emergencies in the Great Outdoors

- Assessing the Situation: Begin by evaluating the severity of the injury or illness. Is the situation life-threatening? Can you safely approach the injured person? Take stock of available resources and personnel.

- Basic Life Support: Ensure the injured person has an open airway and is breathing. If necessary, initiate cardiopulmonary resuscitation (CPR) following the protocols you've learned. Remember that wilderness CPR may require longer duration efforts due to delayed access to medical facilities.

- Stopping Severe Bleeding: Control bleeding by applying direct pressure to the wound with a sterile dressing or clothing. Elevate the injured area if possible. Use tourniquets only as a last resort when bleeding cannot be controlled by other means.

- Fractures and Splinting: In wilderness situations, splinting fractured bones can help stabilize injuries. Use available materials such as branches, trekking poles, or clothing to immobilize the injured limb.

Dealing with Environmental Hazards

- Hypothermia: Hypothermia is a common outdoor threat. Keep affected individuals warm by insulating them from the ground and wind. Use body heat, if necessary, by sharing body warmth. Drink warm, non-alcoholic, non-caffeinated fluids.

- Heat-Related Illnesses: Recognize the signs of heat exhaustion and heatstroke. Move the person to a cooler place, hydrate them, and cool their body using water and shade.

- Dehydration: Stay well-hydrated by drinking regularly, even if you don't feel thirsty. Consume electrolyte-rich foods or solutions to replenish lost minerals.

Utilizing Natural Resources for Survival

- Wilderness Medicine Kit: Assemble a wilderness-specific first aid kit with essentials like sterile dressings, adhesive tape, pain relievers, antiseptics, and personal medications. Include items for treating outdoor-specific injuries like blisters and insect stings.

- Edible and Medicinal Plants: Familiarize yourself with the local flora and fauna, especially plants with medicinal properties and those suitable for consumption. Some common examples include plantain for wounds, willow bark for pain relief (natural aspirin), and pine needles for making vitamin C-rich tea.

- Water Sources: Knowing how to purify water from natural sources is vital. Carry water purification tablets or a portable water filter. In a pinch, boiling water for at least one minute can make it safe to drink.

- Wilderness Navigation: Having map-reading and navigational skills can prevent getting lost in the wilderness. A GPS device and compass are valuable tools, but knowing how to navigate using natural landmarks is equally important.

- Wilderness Communication: Carry a satellite communication device or a personal locator beacon (PLB) in case of emergencies. These devices can summon help when all else fails.

Remember that prevention is the best medicine in the wilderness. Adequate planning, sharing your itinerary with others, and staying informed about local conditions and hazards can go a long way in ensuring a safe outdoor adventure. Additionally, consider enrolling in a wilderness first aid course to gain hands-on experience and confidence in handling medical emergencies in remote settings.

By mastering wilderness first aid skills and preparing for outdoor contingencies, you can enjoy the beauty of the natural world with greater peace of mind, knowing you have the knowledge and tools to respond effectively to unexpected challenges.

CHAPTER 5: MEDICAL EMERGENCIES

Emergencies can happen at any time and in any place, often when you least expect them. Being prepared to identify, respond to, and manage medical emergencies is an essential skill for anyone interested in survival medicine and first aid. In this chapter, we will explore the critical aspects of handling various medical emergencies, including common health crises, allergies, heart attacks, strokes, and the responsible administration of medications.

Identifying and Addressing Common Health Crises

Emergencies come in various forms, and recognizing the signs and symptoms can be a lifesaver. Whether you are in a remote wilderness setting or facing an urban crisis, understanding how to identify and address common health crises is crucial. Some of these include:

- Traumatic Injuries: This includes injuries like cuts, fractures, sprains, and dislocations. Proper wound care, immobilization techniques, and improvised splints can help manage these issues effectively.
- Bleeding: Severe bleeding can be life-threatening. Learn how to control bleeding by applying pressure, using tourniquets (only when necessary), and packing wounds with dressings or materials at hand.
- Burns: Burns can range from minor to severe. Know how to differentiate between first, second, and third-degree burns and provide appropriate treatment. Cool running water is

often the best immediate remedy for minor burns.

- Seizures: Individuals with certain medical conditions may experience seizures. Learn how to protect them from injury during a seizure and provide reassurance afterward.
- Choking: The Heimlich maneuver or abdominal thrusts can be lifesaving when someone is choking on a foreign object. Recognize the signs of choking and act swiftly.

Dealing with Allergies, Heart Attacks, and Strokes

- Allergic Reactions: Allergies can range from mild skin rashes to severe anaphylaxis. Learn to recognize the signs, such as hives, swelling, difficulty breathing, and a drop in blood pressure. Administer epinephrine if available and seek immediate medical help for severe allergic reactions.

- Heart Attacks: Recognize symptoms like chest pain or discomfort, shortness of breath, nausea, lightheadedness, and pain radiating down the arm or jaw. If someone is experiencing a heart attack, call emergency services immediately and assist with aspirin administration if advised by medical professionals.

- Strokes: Strokes can cause sudden numbness, weakness, confusion, trouble speaking, or a severe headache. Use the FAST (Face, Arms, Speech, Time) acronym to identify stroke symptoms quickly. Seek emergency medical attention immediately if someone is having a stroke.

Administering Medications When Necessary

- Epinephrine (EpiPen): Individuals with severe allergies may carry an epinephrine auto-injector, such as an EpiPen. Follow the instructions for administration if someone experiences a severe allergic reaction. Always seek immediate medical help afterward.

- Aspirin: In the event of a suspected heart attack, emergency medical services may recommend chewing aspirin to help thin the blood and reduce the risk of blood clots. Provide aspirin to the person if advised by medical professionals.

- Prescription Medications: If you are caring for someone with known medical conditions, ensure they have access to their prescribed medications, and help them take the correct doses as needed.

- Nitroglycerin: Some individuals with heart conditions carry nitroglycerin tablets or spray for angina (chest pain). If someone is experiencing chest pain and has nitroglycerin, assist them in taking the medication as prescribed.

- Blood-Thinning Medications: If someone on blood-thinning medications experiences uncontrolled bleeding, apply pressure to the wound and seek immediate medical attention.

Understanding how to manage these medical emergencies can make a significant difference in the outcome. While this chapter provides guidance, always remember that professional medical help is essential. When in doubt, call emergency services promptly. Your ability to recognize the signs and take prompt action can be invaluable in a crisis.

CHAPTER 6: INJURIES AND TRAUMA

Accidents and injuries can happen at any time and in any place. Being prepared to provide first aid for injuries and trauma is a valuable skill that can make a significant difference in the outcome. This chapter covers essential techniques for wound care and infection prevention, stopping severe bleeding, and handling head injuries and spinal trauma.

Techniques for Wound Care and Infection Prevention

- Assessing the Wound: Begin by assessing the wound's size, depth, and severity. Look for foreign objects or debris that may be embedded in the wound.

- Cleaning the Wound: Clean the wound gently with a mild soap and clean, lukewarm water. Avoid using hydrogen peroxide or alcohol, as they can damage tissue. If possible, irrigate the wound with a sterile saline solution.

- Antiseptic Application: Apply an antiseptic ointment or solution to the wound to prevent infection. Use a sterile dressing or bandage to cover the wound and keep it clean.

- Dressing Changes: Change the dressing regularly, following the recommended schedule for the type of wound. Look for signs of infection, such as increased redness, swelling, or pus.

- Tetanus Prevention: For puncture wounds, deep cuts, or wounds from dirty objects, ensure that the injured person's tetanus vaccination is up to date. Tetanus is a potentially serious bacterial infection that can result from contaminated wounds.

Stopping Severe Bleeding

- Direct Pressure: Apply direct pressure to the bleeding wound using a clean cloth, gauze, or your hand. Maintain pressure for at least 10-15 minutes or until bleeding stops.
- Elevation: If possible, elevate the bleeding limb above heart level. This can help reduce blood flow to the area and control bleeding.
- Tourniquet Use: Tourniquets should only be used as a last resort when life-threatening bleeding cannot be controlled by other means. Apply a tourniquet above the bleeding site, ensuring it is tight enough to stop the bleeding but not so tight that it causes additional

damage. Note the time the tourniquet was applied and seek professional medical help immediately.

Handling Head Injuries and Spinal Trauma

- Head Injuries: Head injuries can range from mild concussions to severe traumatic brain injuries. If someone experiences a head injury, check for signs of concussion, such as confusion, loss of consciousness, or memory problems. Keep the person still and seek medical evaluation for any significant head trauma.

- Spinal Trauma: Suspected spinal injuries require extreme caution. If you suspect a spinal injury, keep the injured person still and immobilize the head and neck by using improvised cervical collars or manually stabilizing the head. Do not move the person unless it is absolutely necessary to prevent further injury.

- Transport Safely: When transporting an individual with a suspected head or spinal injury, use a rigid backboard or similar equipment to maintain immobilization. Ensure proper support for the head and neck during transport.

- Concussion Recognition: Recognizing and responding to concussions is crucial. If someone experiences a blow to the head, monitor them for signs of concussion and seek medical evaluation if necessary. Rest and cognitive rest are often recommended during concussion recovery.

Remember that providing first aid for injuries and trauma is not a substitute for professional medical care. In cases of severe bleeding, head injuries, or suspected spinal trauma, always seek immediate medical attention. Your actions can help stabilize the injured person and prevent complications while awaiting professional help. Additionally, stay up-to-date with first aid training and regularly review and refresh your knowledge to be prepared for unexpected situations.

Chapter 7: Survival Medicine for Specific Environments

Survival medicine isn't a one-size-fits-all practice. It varies depending on the environment you find yourself in. Whether you're in an urban jungle, the remote wilderness, or traveling to unfamiliar places, each setting presents unique medical challenges. In this chapter, we'll explore how to prepare for and cope with medical emergencies in urban, rural, and wilderness environments, as well as how to navigate medical crises while traveling.

Urban Survival Medicine

In urban areas, help is often just a phone call away, but you may still encounter challenges during emergencies.

- Traffic and Access: Consider how traffic and crowded streets can impede the arrival of emergency services. Know alternative routes and, if possible, learn basic urban navigation skills.

- First Aid in High-Rise Buildings: In high-rise buildings, access to medical help may be delayed. Learn how to manage injuries, administer first aid, and safely transport injured individuals in confined spaces.

- Hygiene and Sanitation: Urban survival often means dealing with overcrowded conditions. Be prepared to address sanitation and hygiene issues to prevent the spread of disease.

Rural Survival Medicine

Rural areas may have fewer resources and longer response times from emergency services.

- Remote Location Awareness: Familiarize yourself with your surroundings. Know the locations of nearby medical facilities, emergency contacts, and potential hazards unique to rural areas.
- Animal and Insect Bites: In rural settings, encounters with wildlife and insects are more common. Learn how to manage bites and stings and recognize signs of infections like Lyme disease.
- Water Safety: Understand the safety of local water sources. In rural areas, clean water

sources may be limited, and waterborne illnesses are a concern.

Wilderness Survival Medicine

The wilderness offers unmatched beauty but comes with its own set of medical challenges.

- Extended Isolation: Wilderness settings can mean days or weeks without access to medical help. Learn how to stabilize injuries and illnesses until rescue is possible.
- Hypothermia and Hyperthermia: Understand the dangers of extreme temperatures. Learn how to prevent and treat hypothermia (extreme cold) and hyperthermia (extreme heat) in the wilderness.
- Navigation and Communication: Carry navigation tools like maps and compasses, and know how to use them. Invest in a satellite

communication device or personal locator beacon (PLB) for emergencies.

Travel Medicine

Traveling exposes you to unfamiliar environments, healthcare systems, and potential health risks.

- Pre-Travel Planning: Research your destination's health risks and vaccination requirements. Pack a well-equipped travel medical kit containing essentials for common ailments and injuries.
- Food and Water Safety: Be cautious of the food and water you consume while traveling. Follow safe food handling practices and use water purification methods when needed.
- Local Healthcare Knowledge: Familiarize yourself with local healthcare facilities and how

to access them. Consider purchasing travel insurance that covers medical emergencies.

By recognizing the unique challenges and preparations required in urban, rural, wilderness, and travel environments, you can enhance your ability to respond effectively to medical crises. Tailor your survival medicine knowledge and supplies to fit the specific demands of each setting, ensuring that you're well-prepared no matter where you find yourself. Remember that while these skills are valuable, seeking professional medical help is always the top priority in emergencies.

Chapter 8: Self-Care and Mental Resilience

Survival situations often test not only our physical abilities but also our mental strength. In this chapter, we'll delve into the crucial aspects of self-care and mental resilience that can make a significant difference in your ability to survive and thrive during challenging circumstances. We'll explore how maintaining mental well-being and practicing self-care routines can be just as essential as physical survival skills in the face of adversity.

Managing Stress and Anxiety in Survival Situations

- Understanding Stress Responses: Stress is a natural reaction to challenging situations. Learn to recognize the physical and emotional signs of stress, such as increased heart rate or irritability.

- Breathing and Relaxation Techniques: Deep breathing and relaxation exercises can help reduce stress and anxiety. Practice these techniques regularly to stay calm under pressure.

- Positive Self-Talk: Train your mind to focus on positive thoughts. Replace negative self-talk with affirmations and reminders of your strengths.

- Mindfulness and Grounding: Mindfulness practices can help you stay present and reduce feelings of panic. Grounding exercises, like focusing on your senses, can anchor you in the moment.

Prioritizing Self-Care for Physical and Mental Well-Being

- Adequate Rest: Lack of sleep can impair decision-making and weaken your resilience. Prioritize rest when possible, and establish sleep routines even in challenging environments.

- Nutrition and Hydration: Proper nutrition and staying hydrated are essential for mental clarity and physical stamina. Learn to identify edible plants and sources of clean water in the wild.

- Maintaining Personal Hygiene: Basic hygiene practices, such as washing hands and staying clean, are vital for preventing illness and maintaining morale.

- Social Connection: Human interaction is crucial for mental well-being. Foster connections with others in your survival group or reach out to family and friends when possible.

- Mindful Practices: Incorporate mindfulness techniques, such as meditation or journaling, to manage stress and maintain mental resilience.

Fostering Resilience and Adaptability

- Embrace Change: Survival situations often require adapting to rapidly changing circumstances. Cultivate a flexible mindset that embraces change and seeks solutions.

- Problem-Solving Skills: Develop your problem-solving skills by breaking down challenges into manageable steps. Stay calm, think critically, and prioritize tasks.

- Learn from Experience: Reflect on past survival experiences, if any, and learn from both successes and mistakes. This knowledge can enhance your resilience.

- Set Realistic Goals: Set achievable short-term and long-term goals. Celebrate small victories to boost morale and maintain a sense of purpose.
- Maintain Hope: Hope is a powerful motivator. Focus on your vision of survival and the positive outcomes you wish to achieve.
- Stay Informed: Gather information about your environment and adapt your survival strategies accordingly. Knowledge is a valuable asset in any survival situation.

Remember that self-care isn't a luxury but a necessity for survival. By effectively managing stress, prioritizing self-care practices, and fostering mental resilience and adaptability, you enhance your ability to endure and overcome the challenges that come your way during survival situations. Ultimately, your mental state can be as critical as your physical skills when it comes to staying safe and thriving in the face of adversity, ensuring your overall well-being during trying times.

CHAPTER 9: COMMUNICATING IN CRISIS

In a survival or emergency situation, effective communication can mean the difference between life and death. Whether you're conveying critical medical information, seeking assistance from responders, or maintaining contact with your survival group, clear and accurate communication is paramount.

Effective Communication with Responders

- Stay Calm and Clear: When interacting with emergency responders or professionals, it's essential to stay calm and articulate. Clearly describe the situation, injuries, or medical conditions.

- Use Recognized Signals: In some survival situations, recognized signals or distress codes can help convey urgency or need for assistance. Learn and use these signals when appropriate.

- Keep It Simple: Complex information can be challenging to convey in high-stress situations. Stick to the most critical details, and avoid unnecessary jargon or technical terms.

- Follow Instructions: If responders or authorities provide instructions, follow them carefully. This ensures your safety and the safety of those around you.

Using Emergency Communication Devices

- Two-Way Radios: Two-way radios or walkie-talkies are valuable for maintaining communication within your survival group or with authorities if you're in an area with coverage. Ensure batteries are charged and carry spares.

- Emergency Beacons: Personal locator beacons (PLBs) or satellite messengers can be lifesavers. Activate them in dire situations to signal for help and provide your GPS coordinates.

- Cell Phones: While cell phone coverage can be limited in remote areas, carry a charged phone and try to reach emergency services if possible. Keep in mind that GPS may not work without cellular coverage.

- Signal Mirrors and Whistles: In wilderness scenarios, signal mirrors and whistles can help attract attention from a distance. Practice using them effectively.

Conveying Medical Information Accurately

- Prepare a Medical History: Before embarking on any outdoor or survival adventure, compile a list of your group's medical histories, allergies, and any pre-existing conditions. Keep this information readily accessible.

- Use Clear Language: When describing medical issues, use plain and straightforward language. Avoid medical jargon that responders may not understand.

- Include Medications: Provide details about any medications taken by members of your group, including dosage and frequency.

- Allergies and Sensitivities: Highlight any allergies, sensitivities, or adverse reactions to specific substances. This information can be critical for medical treatment.

- Prioritize Injuries: When providing medical information, prioritize injuries or conditions based on severity. This helps responders assess the situation and allocate resources effectively.
- Update as Needed: If the medical condition of anyone in your group changes, update the information provided to responders promptly.
- Establish a Communication Plan: In your group, establish a communication plan that includes designated communication times and protocols. Ensure everyone knows how to use the communication devices.

Remember that effective communication is a skill that can be honed through practice and training. In survival situations, it's vital to convey information accurately and efficiently. Whether you're seeking assistance from responders, communicating with your survival group, or conveying critical medical information, the ability to articulate your needs can significantly impact the outcome of the situation.

CHAPTER 10: LONG-TERM SURVIVAL MEDICINE

When faced with a long-term survival scenario, ensuring the health and well-being of yourself and your group becomes a more complex challenge. Sustaining health and hygiene over extended periods, utilizing natural remedies and herbal medicine, and addressing nutritional needs are crucial aspects of long-term survival medicine.

Sustaining Health and Hygiene over Extended Periods

- Water Purification: Access to clean water is paramount. Invest in a reliable water purification system, and know how to source, filter, and purify water from natural sources.

- Sanitation: Proper waste disposal and maintaining personal hygiene are essential to prevent illness. Establish a sanitation system for your camp and adhere to strict hygiene practices.

- Injury Prevention: In long-term survival, preventing injuries takes on added importance. Stay vigilant, maintain a safe camp environment, and practice situational awareness.

Utilizing Natural Remedies and Herbal Medicine

- Wild Plant Identification: Learn to identify local plants with medicinal properties. Herbal remedies can be invaluable for treating common ailments, injuries, and maintaining health.

- Herbal First Aid Kit: Create an herbal first aid kit with essential items like comfrey for wound healing, yarrow for fever reduction, and chamomile for relaxation and sleep.
- Teas and Tinctures: Understand the preparation of herbal teas and tinctures. These can provide relief from various health issues and enhance overall well-being.

Addressing Nutritional Needs during Survival Scenarios

- Foraging for Wild Edibles: Acquire knowledge of edible plants in your region. Foraging for wild edibles can supplement your diet with essential nutrients.

- Hunting and Fishing: Develop hunting and fishing skills to secure protein sources. Snares, traps, and fishing lines should be part of your survival gear.

- Food Preservation: Learn food preservation techniques like smoking, drying, or fermenting to extend the shelf life of perishables.

- Nutritional Balance: Strive for a balanced diet. Pay attention to the intake of macronutrients (carbohydrates, proteins, fats) and micronutrients (vitamins and minerals).

- Emergency Rations: Include long-lasting, high-calorie emergency rations in your supplies. These are valuable for times when food is scarce.

- Supplements: Consider carrying essential vitamins and minerals in supplement form to prevent deficiencies.

- Water Retention: In survival scenarios, water may be limited. Conserve water through efficient cooking methods and minimize unnecessary water loss.

CHAPTER 11: COMMUNITY AND MUTUAL AID

In times of crisis, the importance of community and mutual aid cannot be overstated. When facing challenging situations or disasters, individuals and groups who come together to support one another often fare better than those who go it alone. This chapter explores the power of collaboration during crises, building a support network for survival, and the significance of sharing knowledge and resources.

The Power of Collaboration During Crises

- Strength in Numbers: Communities can achieve more collectively than individuals can on their own. During emergencies, the combined skills, resources, and efforts of a group can enhance resilience and survival.

- Emotional Support: Loneliness and isolation can exacerbate stress and anxiety in challenging situations. Being part of a community provides emotional support and a sense of belonging, helping individuals cope with adversity.

- Diverse Skillsets: Communities often comprise individuals with diverse skillsets. This diversity allows for a broader range of expertise, from medical knowledge to construction skills, which can be invaluable in various survival scenarios.

Building a Support Network for Survival

- Community Building: Start by connecting with neighbors, friends, or local organizations that share an interest in emergency preparedness and survival. Online forums and social media groups can be valuable for finding like-minded individuals.

- Regular Training: Organize training sessions and workshops to build skills together. This might include first aid and medical training, disaster response drills, and wilderness survival lessons.

- Resource Sharing: Create a shared resource pool within your community. This could include communal supplies like food, water, medical kits, and tools.

- Communication Plan: Develop a communication plan that ensures everyone in the group can stay in touch during an emergency. This might involve designated meeting points, communication apps, or two-way radios.

Sharing Knowledge and Resources

- Education and Training: Share your knowledge and skills with others, and encourage them to do the same. Knowledge about survival medicine, foraging, and other essential skills should be disseminated within the community.
- Resource Allocation: Establish fair and transparent systems for resource allocation within the group. Decisions about resource distribution should be based on need and contribution.
- Community Roles: Define roles and responsibilities within the community. This

ensures that everyone knows what is expected of them and can contribute effectively to the group's well-being.

- Resilience in Numbers: The more self-sufficient individuals are within the community, the less they rely on external assistance. This self-reliance increases overall resilience.

- Mental Health Support: Recognize the psychological toll that survival situations can take. Provide emotional support and encourage open communication to help community members cope with stress.

By fostering a sense of community and mutual aid, individuals and groups can significantly improve their chances of survival during emergencies. Remember that collaboration not only enhances physical resources but also provides emotional support and a shared sense of purpose. As you build your community and develop these relationships, you are investing in a network that can make all the difference when the unexpected occurs. In times of crisis, the bonds you create can be a lifeline, ensuring that no one faces adversity alone.

CHAPTER 12: PREPARING FOR THE UNKNOWN

In a world that seems increasingly unpredictable, preparing for the unknown becomes a vital aspect of survival medicine and first aid. This chapter delves into the importance of recognizing the unpredictability of emergencies, the need for constant updates to your survival skills, and the significance of encouraging others to prioritize survival education.

Recognizing the Unpredictability of Emergencies

- Nature's Unpredictability: Natural disasters such as earthquakes, hurricanes, and wildfires can strike without warning. It's crucial to understand that nature operates on its own timeline, and emergencies can occur at any moment.

- Human-Caused Disasters: Beyond natural disasters, human-caused emergencies like industrial accidents, terrorism, and civil unrest can be equally unpredictable. These situations often arise suddenly, leaving little time for preparation.

- Global Health Crises: Recent global health crises have highlighted the need to prepare for pandemics. The rapid spread of diseases like COVID-19 emphasizes the importance of being ready for unexpected health emergencies.

Constantly Updating Your Survival Skills

- Lifelong Learning: Survival medicine and first aid are fields that are constantly evolving. New techniques, technologies, and research emerge regularly. It's essential to commit to lifelong learning and stay up-to-date with the latest developments.

- Regular Practice: Like any skill, survival skills require regular practice to maintain proficiency. Review and practice your first aid and survival techniques periodically, ensuring that muscle memory and knowledge stay sharp.

- Adaptability: The ability to adapt to new situations is crucial. Understand that each emergency is unique, and your survival strategies may need to be adjusted accordingly. Flexibility and adaptability are key.

- Networking: Connect with like-minded individuals and survival experts to share knowledge and experiences. Attend workshops, seminars, and training sessions to expand your skill set and stay informed.

Encouraging Others to Prioritize Survival Education

- Community Workshops: Organize workshops and training sessions in your community to encourage others to prioritize survival education. Cover essential topics such as basic first aid, emergency preparedness, and self-sufficiency.

- Family Preparedness: Advocate for family preparedness by discussing the importance of having an emergency plan and adequate supplies. Encourage loved ones to participate in training and preparation efforts.

- Educational Initiatives: Support educational initiatives in schools and communities to introduce survival and first aid education at an early age. This can foster a culture of preparedness.

- Leading by Example: Lead by example and share your own preparedness journey. Demonstrating your commitment to survival education can inspire others to follow suit.

- Online Resources: Utilize online platforms, social media, and blogs to share valuable information about survival medicine and first aid. Engage with communities interested in emergency preparedness to broaden your reach.

By recognizing the unpredictability of emergencies, continuously updating your survival skills, and encouraging others to prioritize survival education, you contribute to a safer and more prepared society. In a world where the unexpected can happen at any time, your commitment to readiness not only enhances your own survival but also has the potential to save lives and build resilient communities. Remember that preparedness is not a one-time effort but an ongoing journey that evolves with the changing landscape of potential emergencies.